I0503162

HOW TO LIVE WITH PEOPLE AFFECTED WITH MENTAL ILLNESS

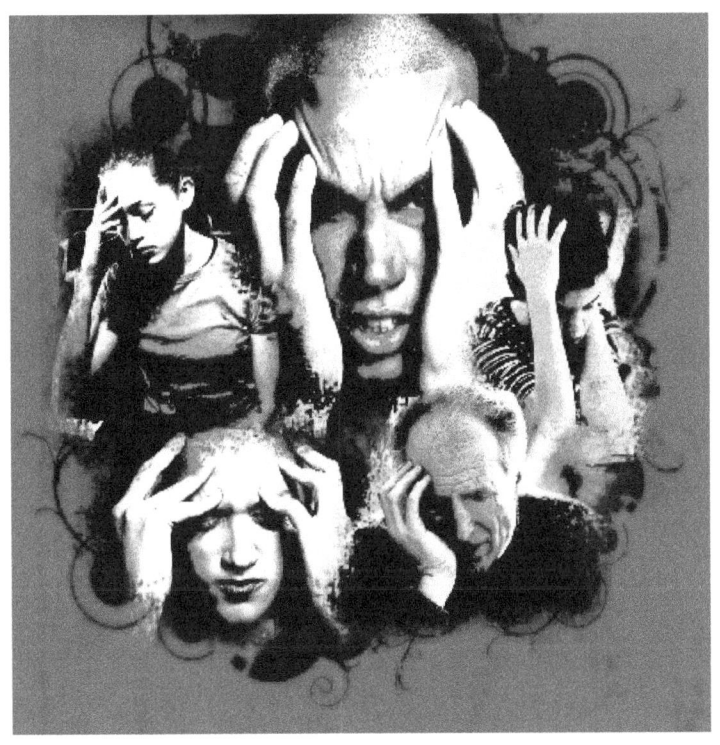

By Patricia A. Carlisle

Introduction

I want to thank you and congratulate you for choosing the book, *"HOW TO LIVE WITH PEOPLE AFFECTED WITH MENTAL ILLNESS"*.

This book contains proven steps and strategies on how to successfully and comfortably live with someone with a mental illness in your home.

Mental illness is stated as any of the various disorders in which a person's thoughts, emotions, or behavior are so abnormal as to cause suffering to himself, herself, or other people, or any other of the various disorders or diseases characterized by abnormal patterns of thought and behavior.

So just talk to the person. You must learn about the illness if the person you care for has been given a diagnosis. This is one of the ways that can help you understand how it affects them, and can help you feel more confident caring for them.

Thanks again for choosing this book, I hope you enjoy it!

TABLE OF CONTENT

Chapter 1

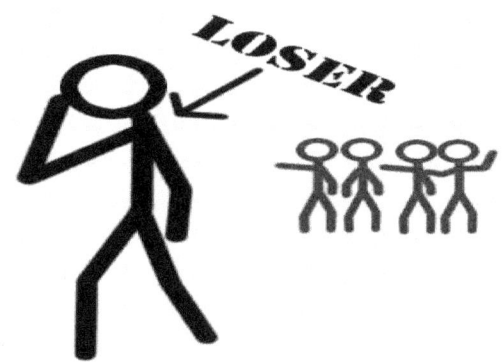

INTRODUCTION

Stigma associated with mental illness and psychiatric treatment, and the discrimination towards people with mental illnesses that frequently results from this, are the main obstacles preventing early and successful treatment. To reduce such stigma, and discrimination towards mentally ill people, and especially those with schizophrenia, the World Psychiatric Association's (WPA) anti stigma programmed 'Open the Doors' is currently being implemented in more than 20 countries.

The programmed has been undertaken in several project centers in Germany. Public information programs and education measures aimed at selected target groups are intended to improve the public's knowledge regarding symptomatolgy, causes and treatment options for schizophrenia. Improved knowledge should in turn reduce prejudice and negative education. Protest and contact are the key elements of anti stigma strategies recommended by the WPA, and various research groups.

These anti stigma strategies include improving psychiatric care, and psycho-education of patients and families, involving patients and family members in all anti stigma activities, including anti stigma education in the training of health care providers, initiating education activities in the general public, and specific target groups, and promoting social and legal action to reduce discrimination.

Mental illness is stated as any of various disorders in which a person 's thoughts, emotions, or behavior are so abnormal, as to cause suffering to himself, herself, or other people, or Any of various disorders or diseases characterized by abnormal patterns of thought and behavior.

Chapter 2

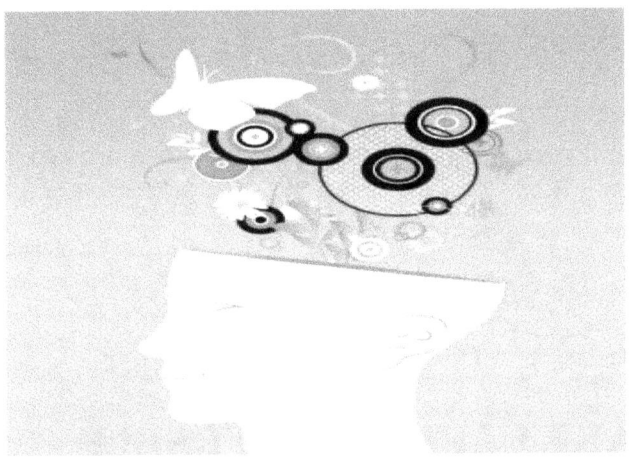

LEARN ABOUT THE ILLNESS

Learn about the illness if the people you care for doctor have given them a diagnosis. This can help you understand how it affects them, and will help you to feel confident caring for them.

You can learn about the illness by going to caregivers groups or services. There you can meet others who have gone through similar experiences, and share support and information. Most areas have caregivers groups or services. You can search online for their contacts.

You can also learn about mental health conditions on trusted websites. The National Health Services (NHS) has reliable information about mental health conditions. You could also buy or borrow a book about the condition from the library.

Talk to the person you are supporting about what symptoms they are having when they are becoming unwell. This will help you to recognize the symptoms when they are becoming unwell in the future. You should talk about what medication they are taking, when they take it, and if they are experiencing any side effects.

Chapter 3

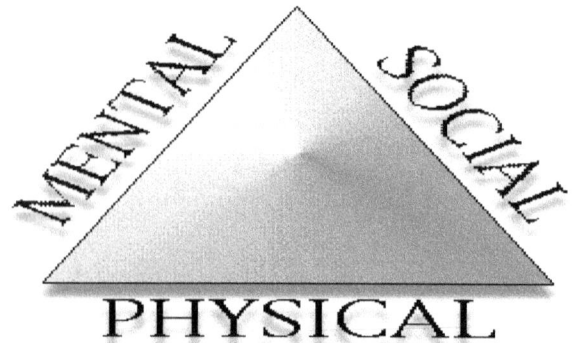

HOW TO TAKE CARE OF YOURSELF EMOTIONALLY AND PRACTICALLY

EMOTINALLY: If you are living with someone with a mental illness, you might find it stressful and difficult. It is important to look after your own health and wellbeing. You can try some of the following things to help you to take care of yourself:

- Understand what you can and can't do as a caregiver.

- Understand what the person you care for can and can't do.

- Give yourself time to do things you want to do, such as a hobby, or leisure activity.

- Try to keep physically active, and have a well balanced diet

- Keep an eye on your own health, and know when you need a break.

- If you are feeling low or stressed, talk to your doctor about this-perhaps counseling, or other treatment will help you.

PRACTICALLY: You may have to organize appointments or meetings if you are supporting someone with a mental illness. There are some things you can do to help with this:

- Keep a diary for their appointments and meetings.

- Keep a diary of medications and times to be taken, checking them off as they are taken.

- Know what benefits you may be entitled to.

- Ask your local council's social services department for a caregiver's assessment. This assessment will help you to see if you need any other services to help you support someone.

- See if there are any local services that can help you with practical support. Your local authority, or social worker may have an updated list of local caregivers groups and services. Check their website or call them.

Chapter 4

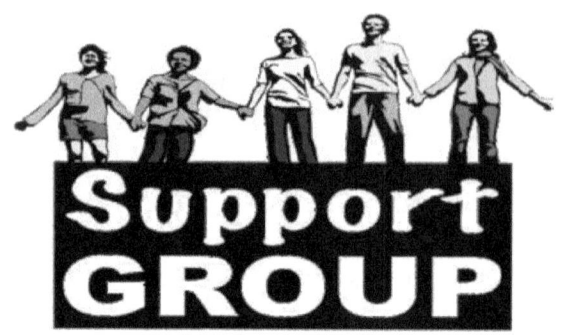

GIVE EMOTIONAL SUPPORT

Offer to listen to the person you are supporting. Listening to someone does not mean you have to say much back to them. Sometimes they may find it helpful to just talk to you about their problems, and to know that you are there to listen.

Do not be afraid to ask them questions about how they are feeling, and listen to their answers. If they are not feeling great, ask if you can do anything to help.

Make sure you do not talk too much so they aren't overwhelmed. This goes a long way to reduce mental illness especially schizophrenia.

Chapter 5

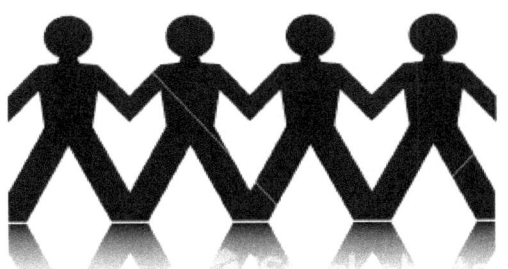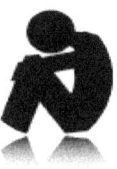

ENCOURAGE THE PERSON TO GET TREATMENT

You may find that the person you are supporting doesn't want to get treatment. This may be because:

- They do not think they need help, and they fell things will get better on their own.

- They are so unwell they do not think treatment will work.

- They do not understand they are not well.

- They are scared of what will happen to them if they tell their doctor how they feel.

- They are worried what other people might think.

- They are worried it will affect their job or studies.

- They feel hopeless.

If the person you care for doesn't want to get help, it can be very frustrating. Nobody can force someone else to get medical treatment unless they are in the hospital under the Mental Health Act (sometimes called being 'sectioned'), or on a 'community treatment order'.

It may help if you offer to go to an appointment with them, and support them during that appointment. If they don't want you to go to the appointment you could offer to wait outside, or in the waiting area.

If someone you care for does not want to get help you could try to:

- Talk to them about how they feel.

- Ask them why they do not want to get help.

- Explain that you are worried because they seem upset, down, stressed or worried, and you want to help them.

- Explain what kind of help they could get.

- Offer to help them talk to their doctor, or offer to talk to their doctor before their appointment.

- Try to convince them they are not crazy.

If the person you are supporting has delusional or paranoid beliefs, they may also feel that other people are plotting against them. This is a very difficult situation to manage, and is common in psychotic conditions such as schizophrenia. It can make things worse if you try to directly challenge the delusions, for example, by saying 'but the doctor is there to help'.

Chapter 6

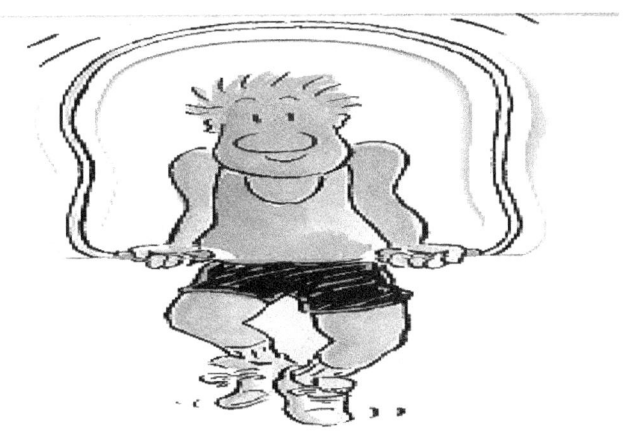

ENCOURAGE THE PERSON TO KEEP ACTIVE

Diet, exercise, and staying active are important for everyone. Staying active with mental illness can be especially important. It can help improve mood, and can help with some of the side effects that medication causes.

You could try to invite the person you care for to go for a walk, swim or to the gym. It can be helpful for you as well to have a routine of getting out and about.

If the person you care for can't leave the house you can ask them to do cleaning around the house, help prepare for meals, or do home exercises. You can get free exercise programs on the internet, or borrow DVDs from your local library. They may not want to do this, and find this to be very boring, but it is important to have some routine, and responsibilities during the day.

An unbalanced diet or eating too much, or not enough can make getting better harder. You can ask your doctor for a healthy diet plan which gives tips and recipes ideas to try out.

Chapter 7

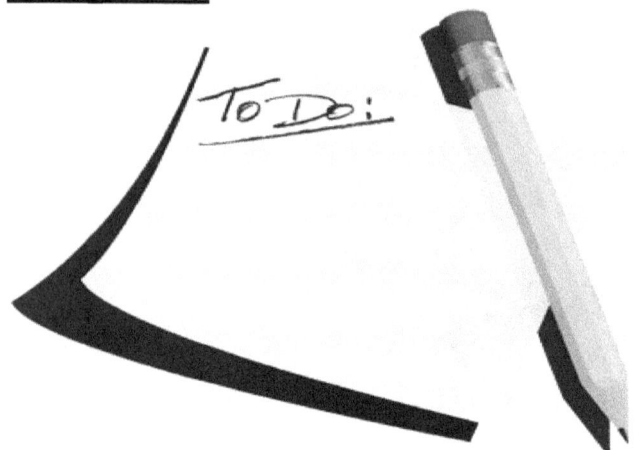

HELP THEM MANAGE WORK AND FINANCES

Some people with mental illnesses will find it difficult to manage their money. For example, when someone with bipolar disorder has a manic episode, they may spend their weekly budget in one day. If the person you care for cannot control their own money, you might want to think about ways to help them.

You could help them manage their own money by:

- Creating a weekly budget.

- Planning what bills need to be paid using a schedule.

- Talking to a money advisory service for further tips.

Having some responsibility outside of the house can be helpful. The person you care for might want to find paid or voluntary work. There are services that help people with mental illnesses to get back into the work force, or do voluntary work. Unfortunately these services are not available across all of the Countries.

Organizations such as Remploy and Shaw Trust, may be able to help and give you options for dealing with someone else's financial affairs, and give you information on work and mental illness.

Chapter 8

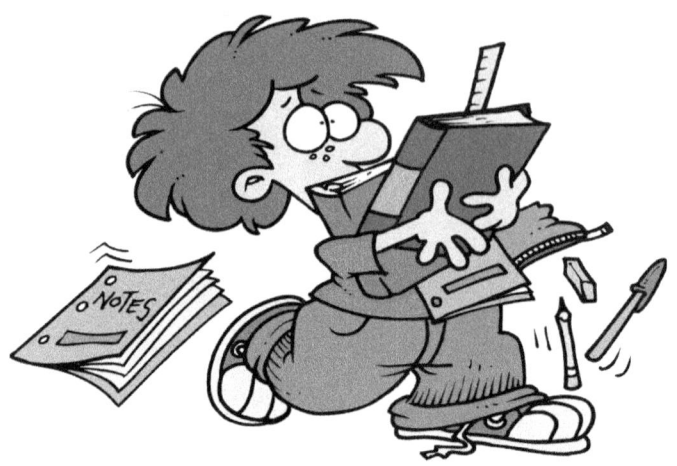

PREPARE YOURSELF FOR DIFFICULT TIMES

By learning as much as you can about the illness and its treatment, and considering what you can reasonably do to support the person. Discuss this with other family members, and the treating health professionals.

If there is a type of care you cannot provide, then discuss with the health professional what arrangements can be made to provide it in some other way. For instances:

Hallucinations

When your family member seems to be hearing voices, or sees things that you do not see, stay calm. Try to distract her or him by asking them to do something, or by engaging them in conversation. If your family member is hearing voices more and more, this may be a sign of relapse.

Encourage your family member to speak with their health professional(s). Do not pretend to see or hear what they hear, but acknowledge what they are hearing, e.g., "I understand you hear another voice even though I don't".

Delusions

Delusions are firmly held false beliefs that can't be changed simply by telling your family member that what they think isn't true. It is pointless to argue with them. Acknowledge that you appreciate that your family member truly believes what they are saying, but don't agree with it.

It is better to help them with the distressing emotions they are feeling rather than to dispel the beliefs. Any delusion is likely to be troubling to your family member and to you. Try to remain calm, and reassure your family member.

It is not uncommon for delusional beliefs to include family members. This type of delusion may be particularly troubling to you, because others may think these beliefs are true. The nature of some delusions may lead you to be concerned about your family member's safety, or well-being.

It may be difficult to know what is true and what is not. As you work this through, it is usually helpful to verify "facts" with others.

Chapter 9

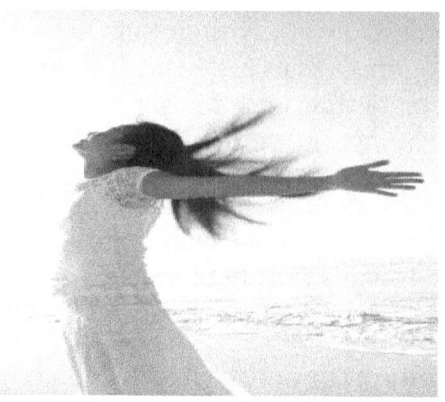

LET THEM ENJOY FUNDAMENTAL FREEDOMS AND BASIC RIGHTS

- All persons have the right to the best available mental health care, which should be part of the health and social care system.

- All persons with mental illness, or who are being treated as such persons, should be treated with humanity and respect for the inherent dignity of the human person.

- All persons with mental illness, or who are being treated as such persons, have the right to protection form economic, sexual and other forms of exploitation, physical, or other abuse and degrading treatment.

- There shall be no discrimination on the grounds of mental illness. "Discrimination" means any distinction, exclusion, or preference that has the effect of nullifying or impairing equal enjoyment of rights. Special measures solely to protect the rights, or secure the advancement, of persons with mental illness shall not be deemed to be discriminatory. Discrimination does not include any distinction, exclusion, or preference undertaken in accordance with the provisions of these principles, and necessary to protect the human rights of a person with a mental illness, or of other individuals.

Every person with a mental illness should have the right to exercise all civil, political, economic, social, and cultural rights as recognized in the Universal Declaration of Human Rights, the International Covenant on Economic, Social and Cultural Rights, the International Covenant on Civil and Political Rights, and the other relevant instruments, such as the Declaration on the Rights of Disabled Persons, and the Body of Principles for the Protection of all Persons under Any form of Detention or Imprisonment.

CONSIDER THE PERSON AS A WHOLE

Remember that they have the same range of personal, emotional and sexual needs as anyone else. Is their physical health being looked after by a doctor? Is alcohol or drugs a problem which needs attention as a solution for their mental illness? Don't think negatively, just begin to see another side of him/her, and carefully help them to become stable.

Chapter 10

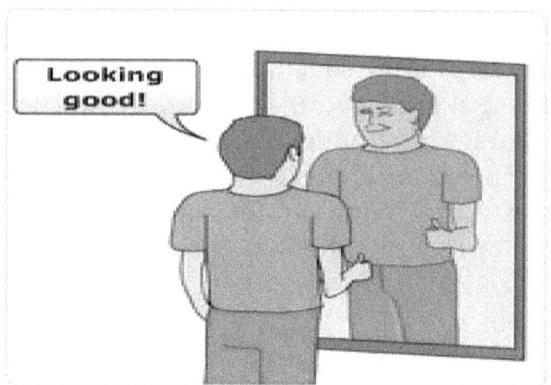

DEVELOPING A PRACTICAL, POSITIVE ATTITUDE

This means: coming to terms with the fact that someone you care for has a mental illness, and that this is likely to have a serious emotional impact on you as well as them. There may be anger because this is happening in your family, confusion, or a sense of loss and grief at how the person has changed because of their illness. It's important to acknowledge, and talk about these feelings.

DEVELOPING A SENSE OF BALANCE

- Acknowledging the effects of the illness on the person and hopes for recovery.

- Wanting to do things to help the person, and encouraging them to be independent.

- Showing you care, and not being over-involved.

- Giving the person your time, and having time for yourself and other family members.

- Encouraging the person to do things, and not being unrealistic and demanding.

Chapter 11

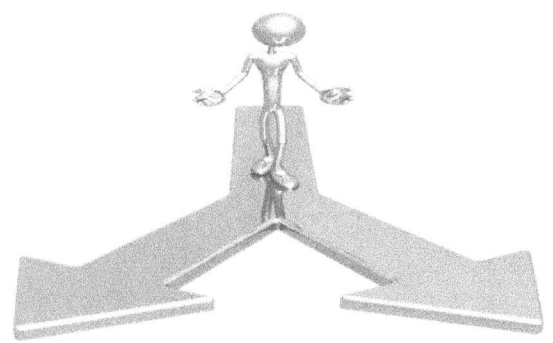

HELP THE PERSON BECOME INDEPENDENT

When you care for someone they can become very dependent on you. Over time the person you care for can rely on you for things they could do themselves. Think about giving them more chances to make decisions, and do things for themselves. Over time they may become more comfortable making decisions for themselves which may take some of the pressure off you.

You can try the following:

- Set up some boundaries. You do this by deciding how much you can do, and how much you want to do. Talk to the person you care for, and tell them what you have decided. Remember, once you set up these boundaries it is important to stick with them.

- Talk about the skills the person you care for needs to focus on and agree on goals. You can agree to show them how to do something, and help them with it for a while until they are confident they can do it alone. An example of this might be doing their laundry themselves, or going to the store.

- If the person you care for has support from a Community Mental Health Team (CMHT), or other mental health services, you could talk to their 'care coordinator' about their care plan. You can ask them what they are doing to help them develop independent living skills. If the person is living on their own you could ask about getting help from an occupational therapist, or floating support.

- You can also encourage the person you support to use a personal budget to pay for services that could improve their day to day life. A personal budget is when social services assess their social care needs. They are then given money which they can choose to spend on services they need. Types of services could include computer classes, or a gym membership. Choosing their own service can improve how they feel about themselves. Some services can also improve confidence, and help to establish a daily routine.

Chapter 12

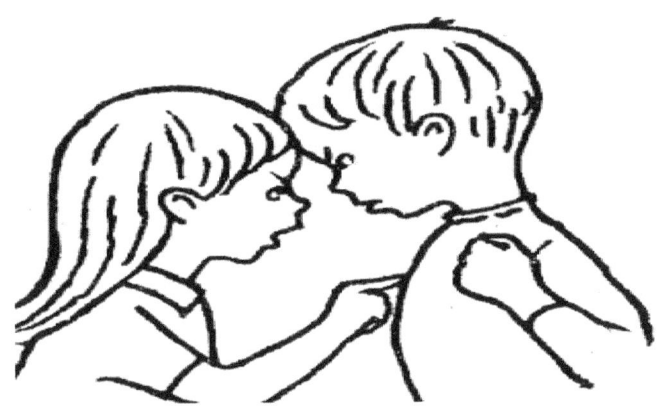

ALWAYS DEFEND THEM WHEN THINGS GET OUT OF HAND

SUICIDAL THOUGHTS:

If the person you are supporting is feeling suicidal you can try some of the following things:

- Ask them about how they are feeling and listen.

- Talk not of any plans they might have.

- Be understanding of their situation.

- Ask them about things that are stopping them from acting on suicidal thoughts. You might be able to find some positive things for them to focus on.

- If all fail, call their doctor, or 911 for help

Conclusion

Thank you again for choosing this book!

I hope this book was able to give you more supportive ideas.

The next step is to be the best caregiver, and enjoy the person and life around you.

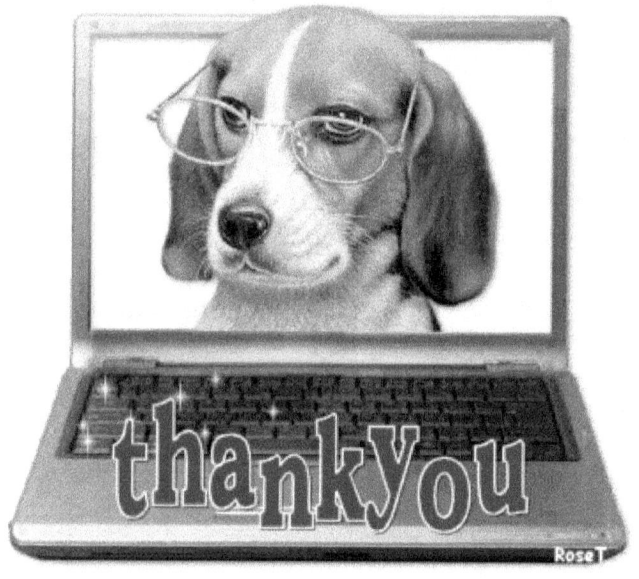

Finally, if you enjoyed this book would you be kind enough to leave a review for this book on Amazon? It'd be greatly appreciated!

Thank you and good luck!

Preview Of 'YOUNG PEOPLE LIVING WITH MENTAL ILLNESS: Learn How to Tell Your Parents'

Chapter 1

RECOGNIZE THE SYMPTOMS

Before telling your parents anything, first of all you need to know yourself. It is impossible to diagnose your own illness and find out exactly what mental disease you have but you can look out for some general symptoms. Try to figure out if your behavior changed in the last period of time.

A sudden change is an extra reason to suspect a mental illness. For example, before you used to be an outgoing person who loved to be surrounded by people. Now you can't stand to be in large groups. You prefer to be alone and you might also have negative thoughts. If those thoughts are turning into suicidal thoughts, you need to tell your parents right away. Together you will go to a doctor and get the urgent help you need. Keeping these things inside can be very dangerous. Some mental illnesses can also cause hallucinations and delusions. You might also have recurring nightmares.

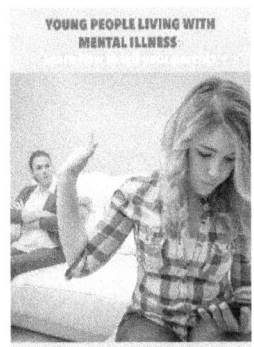 **YOUNG PEOPLE LIVING WITH MENTAL ILLNESS: Learn How To Tell Your Parents**.

Check Out My Other Books

Below you'll find some of my other popular books that are popular on Amazon and Kindle as well. Alternatively, you can visit my author page on Amazon to see other work done by me.

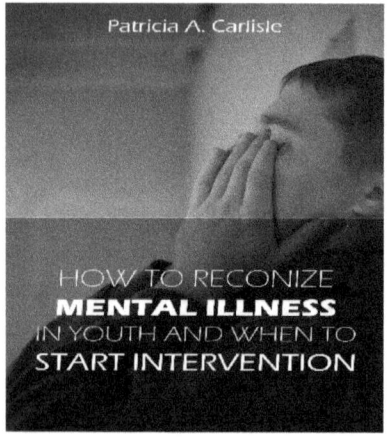

How to Recognize Mental Illness in Youth and When to Start Intervention.

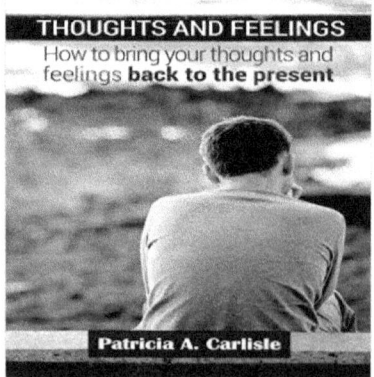

THOUGHTS AND FEELINGS: How to Bring Your Thoughts and Feelings Back to the Present.

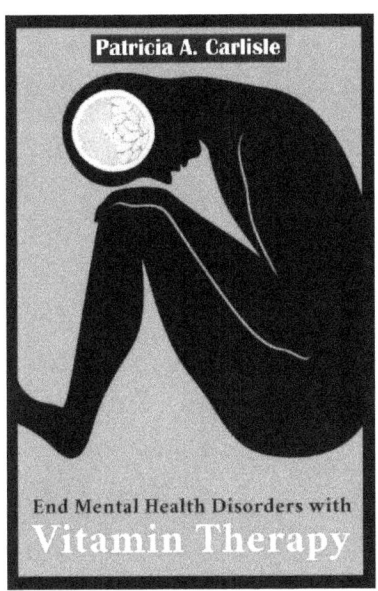

End Mental Disorders with Vitamin Therapy.

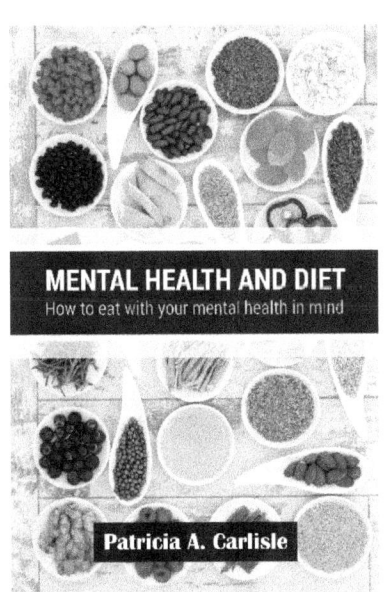

Mental Health and diet: How to eat with your mental health in mind.

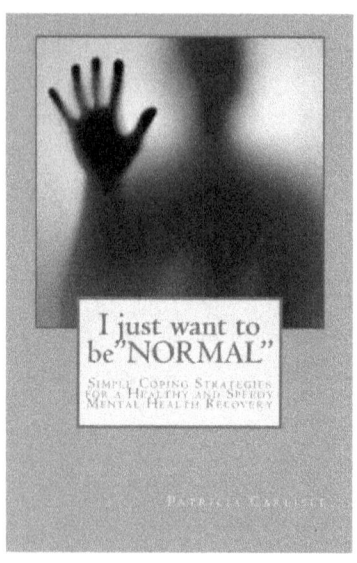

I just want to be"NORMAL": Simple Coping Strategies for a Healthy and Speedy Mental Health Recovery.

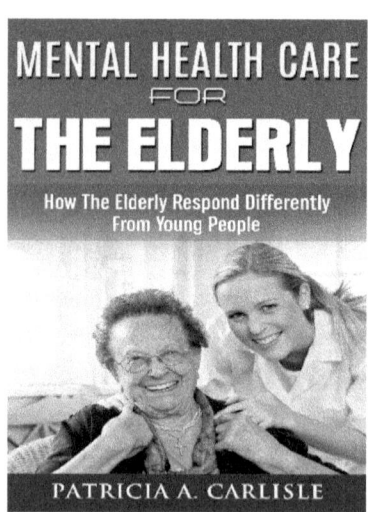

MENTAL HEALTH CARE FOR THE ELDERLY: HOW THE ELDERLY RESPOND DIFFERENTLY FROM YOUNG PEOPLE.

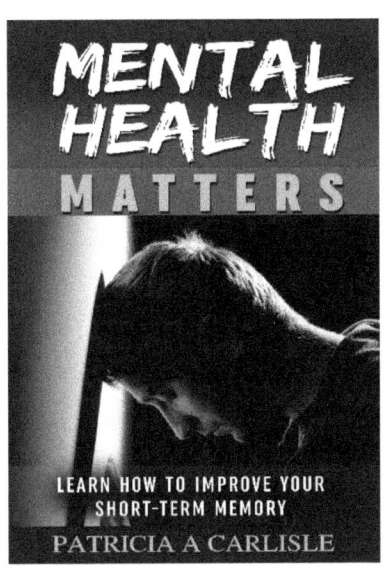

MENTAL HEALTH MATTERS: LEARN HOW TO IMPROVE YOUR SHORT-TERM MEMORY

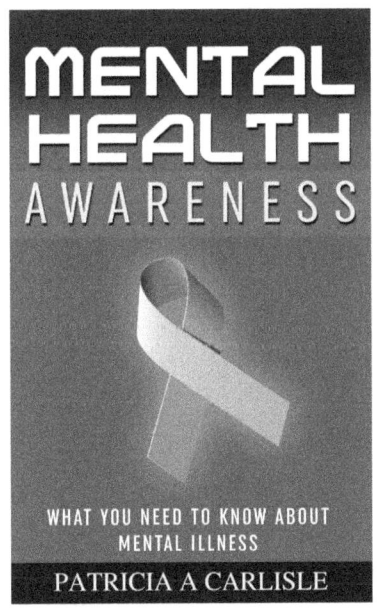

MENTAL HEALTH AWARENESS. WHAT YOU NEED TO KNOW ABOUT MENTAL ILLNESS.

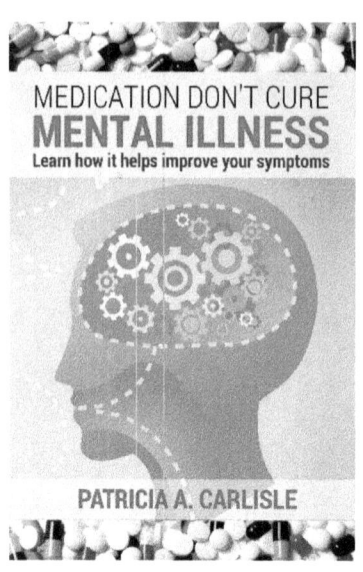

MEDICATION DON'T CURE MENTAL ILLNESS: LEARN HOW IT HELPS IMPROVE YOUR SYMPTOMS.

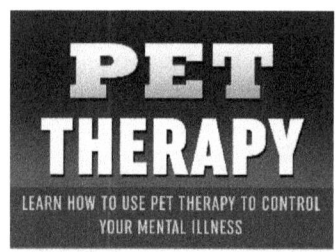

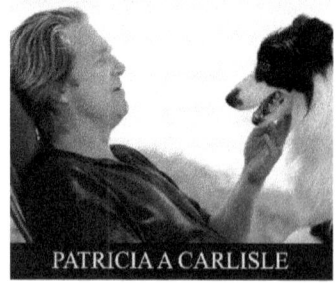

PET THERAPY: LEARN HOW TO USE PET THERAPY TO CONTROL YOUR MENTAL ILLNESS.

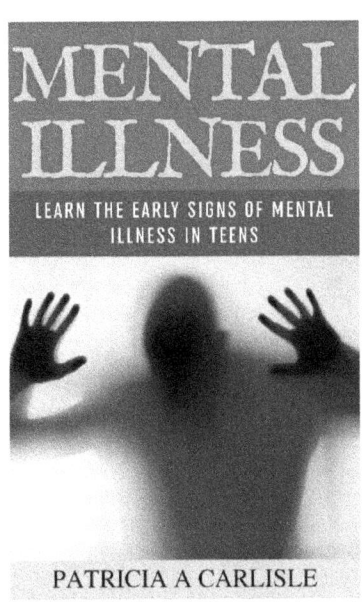

MENTAL ILLNESS: LEARN THE EARLY SIGNS OF
MENTAL ILLNESS IN TEENS.

BONUS: SUBSCRIBE TO THE FREE BOOK

Beginners Guide to Yoga & Meditation

"Stressed out? Do You Feel Like The World Is Crashing Down Around You? Want To Take A Vacation That Will Relax Your Mind, Body And Spirit? Well this Easy To Read Step By Step

E-Book Makes It All Possible!"

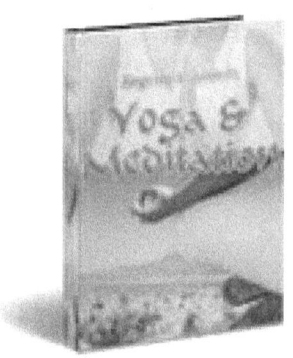

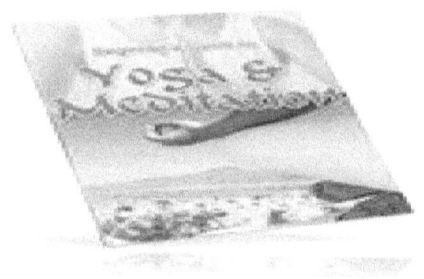

Instructions on how to join our mailing list, and receive a free copy of "Yoga and Meditation" can be found in any of my Kindle eBooks.

NOTES

NOTES

NOTES

NOTES

NOTES

NOTES

NOTES

NOTES

NOTES

NOTES

NOTES

www.ingramcontent.com/pod-product-compliance
Lightning Source LLC
Chambersburg PA
CBHW071013180526
45168CB00003B/1401